MENTAL WEALTH

A GUIDE TO BEING RICH BY SEEKING ENRICHMENT

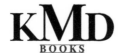

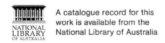
A catalogue record for this work is available from the National Library of Australia

National Library of Australia Catalogue-in-Publication data:

Mental Wealth/Emma Weaver

ISBN:
978-0-6457858-3-8
(Paperback)

Believe in all that you are,
to become all that you can be.

I dedicate this to my three amazing children.
Chloé, Rhys and Amelia.

CONTENTS

CONTRIBUTORS

MENTAL WEALTH

What does wealth mean to you? Is it based on monetary value or your wellbeing, and how do you measure it?

Viktor Frankl, in his book, *Man's Search for Meaning*, mentions research from Johns Hopkins University where participants were asked what was important to them. Sixteen of them said it was to make a lot of money and 78% said their first goal was finding meaning and a purposeful life.

A purposeful life means different things to different people and it's about knowing your way. I recently took part in the seven levels deep exercise, and this has given me so much clarity on my strengths, passion and purpose. Thinking on this, only a small population in the world achieve financial wealth, and the same for mental wealth. Having worked in mental health services for over twenty-two years, I have experienced and learned a lot. Global suicide is at an all-time high; according to the World Health Organization, 800,000 people die by suicide every year – that's one person every forty seconds, the same amount of time it takes to write and send a short message or pay a bill online. The World Health Organization also states that 64 million people are impacted by depression. Your health is truly your wealth and this includes your mental health – I would say even more so. You, and you alone, are responsible for your mental health and wellbeing, and we all have the ability to achieve mental wealth if we truly invest in ourselves.

I believe it's not good enough to just survive with our mental health, we should *thrive* with our mental wealth. Mental wealth is that higher level of mental wellbeing that allows us to achieve our potential, find our passion and purpose, and build resilience to allow us to overcome anything that we are faced with.

In Maslow's theory, we are all aiming or moving towards self-actualisation which is a psychological state of presence with self-acceptance, self-expression and authenticity. This can be achieved when you invest in yourself.

Think of your mental state as your house, you build it bit by bit, you've got good days and bad days, you know what you need to do to build it and setting good foundations is key. The foundations of your wellbeing are thing you practice on a daily basis. These five ways to wellbeing are connect, learn, give, take notice and keep physically active. If you implement these, the public health agency states that it will keep you well, safe and hopefully free from harm in your home. However, this does not make you wealthy. It is what you invest in outside of your home that creates wealth. The same applies for your mental wealth. It is in everyday practices in addition to meeting your basic needs that contribute to this. Set your goals and your intentions develop a plan to action. Then meditation, affirmations, gratitude, raising your energy and your vibration as you deposit money into the bank and let it accumulate, and withdraw it when you need.

The same applies for your mindset. So as with keeping your house in order, you also need to deposit these into a mindset bank so that you can draw on them when you need to. Especially if you have lack of motivation, faced adversity or are hit by the hard knocks of life and we've all had to deal with them. I've known times in my life when I have felt adversity, when I have felt grief, loneliness and pain, and it was in my daily practices that I found strength, courage and resilience. This means that I did not dip as far as I potentially could have because I have achieved mental wealth affirmations discipline in my thoughts.

Creating a healthy mindset is an important factor of the four agreements that are included in all of this. Be impeccable with your word. Do not take anything personally. Do not make assumptions, and always do your best. These raise your level of mindset, adding to your mental wealth. You do not have to achieve this alone. However, to activate mental wealth is to recognise and create a support system around you. I personally am part of an amazing mastermind and also a coaching group of ladies. I invest in myself in all aspects of my life physically, mentally, spiritually and emotionally. Everything is connected in Napoleon Hill's book, *Think and Grow Rich*. He states your body achieves what the mind believes it can. This is paramount. We need to start with our mind as it all comes from within. So who are your five.

It's worth taking a moment to consider this. It is an integral part of creating mental wealth. Your five gold bars swim if you have someone to support you in your spiritual journey. Your wellbeing ambition with your business, someone who keeps you accountable and also supportive with your mindset and motivation. In conclusion, implementing all of these practices in your life will enrich you far more than any amount of money can. Know your five gold bars and it's equally as important to be part of somebody's faith. Open your mindset bank and deposit more than you will ever need to withdraw to maintain optimum wellbeing. Build a stable foundation and invest in your assets. Invest in your mental wealth. Don't just strive for mental health and wellbeing. Thrive for mental wealth.

DO YOU KNOW YOUR FIVE A DAY?

Five always seems to come up – five ways to wellbeing, five fruit and veg a day – but how about we consider our five people a day? They say you are who you spend most of your time with. I am not sure I entirely agree, however, I believe we should be intentional. We all need our needs met and it is important to surround ourselves with the right people; this allows us to thrive emotionally, spiritually and physically in our daily lives.

Do you take time to evaluate who you are surrounded by? Negative energy from people around you can have a deep impact, even if you are not a negative person.

The most important tool at our disposal for living a better life is other people. The people we surround ourselves with are the biggest influence on our behaviour, attitudes and results. Who you are around – what they've got you thinking, saying, doing and becoming.

I often use the acronym SWAAM. Ensuring I am holistically getting my needs met as this leads to ultimate wellbeing and mental wealth.

S is for spiritually. Whatever your belief is, feeling supported and that are you part of something is important. This can be met by a person, a group, online or in-person events.

W is for wellbeing. Who supports you with your wellbeing, is there somewhere you go? Someone who is always there? Have you identified what you need to maintain your wellbeing and surrounded yourself who you need to support this? Have fun with, laugh together, walk with, cry if you need to – these people are gold.

The first A is for ambition. It is important to share your ambition and goals and feel supported either in a group or individually.

The second A is for accountability, someone to keep you on track, give you a gentle nudge to keep going and remind you of your why.

M is for mindset – a space to grow your mind, to sit in your thoughts and tap into your power. This can be a person, a group, book club – whatever meets this need.

It is our responsibility to engage in meaningful interactions with others, and we all have choices when implementing these. We can implement boundaries to ensure that we maintain our wellbeing, which is not always easily done, however, with the right network we can.

As equally as important as having your five people or groups, we need to be part of someone else's five. Be a supporter in whatever way meets their needs. This does not take away from what we need, in fact, it enhances our wellbeing. Helping and working with others can also give us a sense of purpose and feelings of self-worth. Giving our time to others in a constructive way helps us to strengthen our relationships and build new ones, and of course, relationships with others also influence mental wellbeing. Studies have found that acts of kindness are linked to increased feelings of wellbeing. Helping others can also improve our support networks and encourage us to be more active.

So, I ask, are you part of someone's five? Do you know who your five are? Are you intentional about who you choose to spend time with?

YOU DO YOU

SPEAK UP EVEN WHEN YOUR VOICE SHAKES – IT IS GOOD FOR YOUR WELLBEING

In the times we are in, with the digital world being a predominant part of our lives, it is important to stay true to ourselves. By knowing who we are and owning it, we allow for an authentic relationship with ourselves and others. This can be an integral part of our wellbeing. Learning who you are and speaking up for yourself when it is needed can, at times, be hard work – daunting, even – however, what we suppress we repress, meaning it goes inwards and that is unhealthy.

THE BODY KEEPS THE SCORE

There is a fantastic book, *The Body Keeps the Score,* by Bessel van der Kolk, which has allowed me and millions of others to understand that hiding our trauma, challenges and life experiences, not speaking our truth, keeping emotions, thoughts and feelings suppressed has an impact on our physical wellbeing also. We all experience difficulties in our lives, and how we respond has a huge part to play on the impact these events will have on us throughout our lives. Talking about the impact, emotionally and openly about our thoughts around the experience can reduce the impact. Whether it is big or small. Everything we experience shapes us, and creating cultures of sharing these or speaking out at the time can significantly reduce the impact it has on us and generations to come.

Your voice is a tool than can create change in the most adverse situations to help shape a better future for yourself and others. Everyone's voice is important, it can be a superpower when you know how to use it. You never know who you are inspiring when you speak your truth.

You release the inner turmoil when you let it out – and if you feel it is too hard to speak it out loud, say it when you are alone or write it down. Your thoughts and how you are feeling. I use gratitude journals and I also keep a notebook that I mind-dump into as it allows me to release from within. Perhaps read your written words out loud as this can also help.

BENEFITS TO SPEAKING YOUR TRUTH
- You will not feel suppressed.
- Increased confidence.
- Improved self-worth.
- Positive self-esteem.

These are all things that we need for our wellbeing and to improve or health.

NEGATIVES TO NOT USING YOUR VOICE
- Feeling unheard and misunderstood.
- Feeling that your voice is worth less than others.
- Physical stress.

- Low self-esteem.
- Anxiety and/or depression.

Although expressing your emotions may leave you vulnerable – it can be normal to want to hide them – speaking your truth is the best thing for you and your wellbeing.

SHOWING UP FOR YOURSELF

Knowing who you are, setting boundaries and speaking your truth, being authentically you and showing up for yourself is what you are here to do. Own it.

HAPPINESS IS AN INSIDE JOB

Are you familiar with the saying 'never give the key to your happiness to someone else'? Often we feel that others can make us feel good, but taking responsibility for our own happiness is key to creating it and maintaining it too.

We are the holders of our thoughts, feelings and the time and energy we give to people, places and things. So, whether we choose happy, sad or whatever other emotion we feel, it is us that has allowed it.

I believe that happiness is an emotional state – a feeling of joy, wellbeing when you feel gratitude and are mindful in the moment. There are many definitions and a lot to consider, so I encourage you to take time to think about what it is that you are doing or what is happening when you feel happy. I sometimes say it's what you're doing when you lose track of time and do not want it to end – this might be the answer to the question.

Personal freedom from an outside source can allow happiness to flow. A book which speaks about this is *The Four Agreements* by Don

Miguel Ruiz, and his theory on how to obtain personal freedom that I believe can lead to happiness includes some of the following:

BE IMPECCABLE WITH YOUR WORD

Speak with integrity; say only what you mean. Avoid using words to speak against yourself or to gossip about others. This one I feel is true as it means we hold a wonderful energy and do not give time to negativity and remain positive about ourselves and others.

DO NOT TAKE ANYTHING PERSONALLY

Nothing others do is because of you. What others say and do is a projection of their own reality, their own dream. When we realise that we hold the power of our emotions and that others cannot make us think or feel a certain way we understand that it works the same way for them too.

DON'T MAKE ASSUMPTIONS

Find the courage to ask questions and express what you really want. Communicate with others as clearly as you can to avoid misunderstandings, sadness and drama. Imagine how easy life would be if we asked straight up the questions we needed answers to instead of overthinking or guessing, which, let's be honest, rarely ends well. This reduces the drama and creates transparency.

ALWAYS DO YOUR BEST

Your best is going to change from moment to moment. Under circumstances, simply do your best and you will avoid self-judgement, self-abuse and regret.

***

Incorporating these into your daily life and really understanding them can add to your happiness and reduce and sadness, guilt, emotional distress and many other emotions.

When we take ownership of our happiness and implement strategies like the four agreements, the five ways to wellbeing and surrounding ourselves with the right people, it allows us the mental space to create the life we want, know how to create a life of joy and therefore happiness.

FIVE WAYS TO WELLBEING

It is in our daily routine where mental wealth is achieved. These five things are an effective way to achieve and maintain wellbeing.

CONNECT

Connect with others by whatever means you can. We are social beings. The power of human connection allows us to overcome challenges and maintain a state of mental wellbeing. It also decreases physical health risks. It is also important to make sure the right people are around you.

LEARN

Continuous learning helps to keep our mind stimulated and improves our self-esteem which raises our belief in our own abilities. Whatever learning looks like to you – reading, attending college, online courses, audio books and indeed TED Talks or podcasts. The idea is that you keep learning in whatever style you like and at your own pace.

GIVE

We mostly do not give to receive; however, it is the natural way of the world that you receive something in return, and that can simply be the feeling of joy of having given to another person. Giving does not have to be an expensive gift or giving so much of yourself that it is detrimental to your own wellbeing. It can be time – this is one of our most valuable possessions as we can never get it back. By giving someone our time, it is a two-way process – whether a meet-up, a phone call or a video call – giving our most precious asset can reduce feelings of low mood to everyone involved. Giving promotes positive values and life satisfaction. We all have something to give.

TAKE NOTICE

Being aware of the present moment and creating time and space for mindfulness has been proven to help better connect with ourselves and our surroundings. Allowing us to be in the moment away from life's expectations and possibly any stress we may have. Taking notice also can improve our self-awareness, allowing us to focus on our needs, our current thoughts and be present. This can be done on your own or as part of a group. It is so beneficial to our wellbeing and can take time to practice, however, it can have a very positive impact on your wellbeing.

GET ACTIVE

The link between our mental health and physical health has become more evident throughout the years and it is nearly impossible to have one without the other. Maintaining regular physical activity has a huge impact to our wellbeing, mentally and physically. Set yourself physical challenges and goals. They lead to so many positive wellbeing thoughts, self-esteem, increased learning, creativity, productivity and a reduction in anxiety and depression.

It is you, and you alone, that is responsible for your mental health. We all have the ability to achieve mental wealth if we truly put in time and effort. It will not always be easy, but it will be worth it.

***

It is in the actions we take daily that we achieve our desired outcome of wellbeing. If we incorporate the five ways to wellbeing into our daily lives this can lead us to optimum wellbeing – mental wealth, if you like.

Each action can be seen as a deposit into our mental wealth bank, consistently building on our wellbeing reserves creating mindset wealth. Then, when we need it, we can withdraw from it in times of stress, grief, pain, low mood – whatever the challenge is, it is what we have consistently shown up to do daily that will build the resilience and habits that will get us through.

Remember to always reach out for support if you need it.

IT'S ALL IN YOUR DAILY ROUTINE

I have been to many an inspirational day and business confidence course, and each one has had great takeaways. One of the biggest things I hope that you can take away from this book is that it is all about consistency and your daily routine.

Working for over twenty-three years in the mental health space, I recognise that sometimes even getting up and making your bed is an achievement on those tough days. Consistently show up every day and do this, and you have achieved a goal already.

Routines can be implemented easily into your daily life in different levels or aspects:

- *On a personal level:* Think about what activities you engage in on a daily basis. This could mean giving yourself fifteen to twenty minutes a day to enjoy your cup of coffee while reading a book, making time for thirty minutes a day to exercise or giving yourself some time before bed to listen to a podcast. Whatever you choose, make sure you take the time to nurture yourself (whether it's physically, mentally or emotionally) on a daily basis.

Consistency is key. It does not have to be the same activity daily, just ensure you have time for *you.*

- *On a relationship level:* Think about which activities or small things you can do to connect with others. It can be a romantic partner, family member or with a friend on a social level. Make time to talk to someone and hear about their day. Or make a family meal, have a game night once a week or ride bikes as a family on Sundays. Or go on an outing with friends to decompress and destress.

- *On a career/work level:* It doesn't necessarily have to be something to climb up the corporate ladder. It can be something to dig deeper into your professional dreams and goals. Maybe read a book once a month about something in your field of work. Or subscribe to a newsletter that's connected to what you do. Or check LinkedIn once a week and read an interesting article. Or simply network and connect with your colleagues every once in a while to discuss the challenges and opportunities in your professional field.

***

The important thing is to incorporate something in one (or all) of these areas, and make it something you can aspire to or get inspired to accomplish. Whatever it is you'd like to include in your daily life, make sure you write it down in a notebook – I find this helps.

Your day starts the night before, and this is when I write down some tasks I want to achieve the next day and I also get my clothes ready – this is part of my daily routine even though it's for the next day.

TURN YOUR PAIN
INTO PURPOSE

This is a relatively new phrase I have heard lately; at first I wasn't sure about it, however, now I agree. Turn your pain into purpose and share your experience to support others.

We all go through different experiences in our lives, some good and others bad, but we learn from each one. Try to always journal your day and write down your thoughts and feelings on every situation. This is good for several reasons – you can look back and see how far you have come and also remember and pass on the learnings and feelings that you felt at the time so others can benefit from your wisdom and knowledge. Write down your story, what happened to you, how you felt, what you learnt and how you have grown from it. This can be a huge healing experience. Remember to be kind to yourself, this is a process that could make you feel vulnerable.

You can rewrite how you are impacted by it by separating it from you now. Never deny feelings as that's what makes you who you are, but do not let it consume you, and use the energy of the pain to help others.

Feel the feelings, there is healing in the process. Acknowledge that you may have to live with this – however, it does not define you, it can be the making of you. Focus on what is this teaching you or showing you about life.

There have been times in my life when rejection has been redirection. Or when a situation that I am in leads me to understand others better, be less judgemental and become a better person.

In today's world, people relate to lived experiences of others telling their stories – giving hope and showing others the way is very powerful.

When understanding your pain and turning to purpose here are some steps to take:

- Clarify the experience.
- Take a step back and observe.
- Separate the pain from the purpose.
- Learn to trust yourself.

Remember, turning pain into purpose is one of the most powerful healing practices you can commit to. Not only will it change the lives of those you embrace with your strength, wisdom and compassion, it will forever change your life, too. Sometimes all it takes to save someone from hopelessness is another person who's been there and survived.

LIMITING BELIEFS

Limiting beliefs are part of who we are at times. The important thing is to recognise that.

You are experiencing a limiting belief.

Our beliefs are shaped from our childhood.

Our environment, what we were told, what we experienced, maybe what we read and what we believe to be true.

They come in so many different shapes and forms.

They keep us comfortable in our thinking.

In our settings, and allow us to feel that we are confident in knowing these things.

As we grow older, perhaps our beliefs.

Are challenged if we allow them to be.

And I truly believe that this is how we grow. When we feel we cannot do something. Or hear ourselves saying those words, it is what it is.

I think we should pause a moment.

And think, where is that belief coming from? Is it even what we truly believe? Is it something that you haven't inherited?

From your family or the environment that.

You grew up in?

Where has it come from?

Challenge it.

Especially if it is limiting what you are doing, if it is not allowing.

You to reach your potential, if it's.

Making you feel a sense of less or bringing forward imposter syndrome, only you can challenge this. Only you really know where that belief comes from. It can take time.

It took me time as well.

There were certain things in my family that just were the way they were.

And I do believe that with courage, understanding, knowledge and wisdom, we can grow from these things.

There's no right or wrong way.

However, there is your way.

And it does not necessarily have to.

Be the same as everyone else's way. You see, the beauty in life is.

We get to choose. We get to choose how we live, what we do, where we live and who with. What are you going to choose?

Will you choose to challenge those limits.

And beliefs that are maybe holding you.

Back or stopping you from feeling fulfilled.

And reaching your potential?

Write them down, try to work out.

Where they came from, talk about it, put them on the table, work it.

Out and dispel them.

If they are holding you back, they.

Are not serving you a purpose.

Quite often they keep us in our comfort zone.

And, well, we all know nothing grows in comfort zone.

So I challenge you, write down your beliefs.
If they are limiting you, why and how?
And challenge yourself to overcome them.
Learn more and start afresh.

OPPORTUNITIES

Opportunities come to us all in life and we get to choose whether to take them or not. Some people say an opportunity comes to those who are prepared. Opportunities waste no time to those who are ready. However, what happens when preparation meets opportunity?

For example, you'd need to buy a lottery ticket to win the lottery. So you've put yourself in that position, you've created the opportunity. People always say opportunities bring other opportunities. So that is all on how your vibration or where you're putting your energy to.

I quite often talk about always being prepared. Whatever it is that you're doing in life, do it well. Read a lot, know who your tribe are, know what fits your values and what doesn't, and position yourself well. Make sure you're taking action and showing up where you need to. And that is where you find opportunities.

Whether it's in your personal life, your professional life – whatever it is that your goals are and you're aiming for. When you show up, opportunities come your way. Now, this may take time; sometimes it takes work. But if you're ready, when that opportunity comes, you will leave yourself in a position to say yes. Now, do not say yes to everything that comes your way.

Ensure that the opportunities are congruent with your purpose. Does it match your skills, talents and passion? Always be ready. Be prepared. Waiting is not doing anything.

So we need to take action. We need to ensure that the doors are going to open for us.

And if opportunity doesn't come naturally to you, create the opportunity for yourself. After all, the best way to predict your future is to create it. So be aware of what opportunities are for you and what are not. If it feels like they're not coming your way, change your trajectory. Make yourself visible.

Ensure that you are setting the right goals, you've got yourself in the right space, you're talking to the right people. They cannot not come your way.

Not all opportunities are meant for you, so make sure they're the proper ones. Write down what your goals are, what your needs are and how you think you can achieve them. And then just trust that the opportunity will come for you. And most of all, enjoy the journey.

LONLINESS
Loneliness is not the same as being alone.

Loneliness in one aspect of maintaining wellbeing and one that can impact us so much especially here as the dark evenings are coming. Being lonely is not the same as being alone; you can be in a room full of people and still feel lonely.

To be alone means to be physically separated from others, literally on your own. However, with loneliness, you feel emotionally alone and emotionally separate.

There are many different reasons we may experience feelings of loneliness – new job, bereavement, relationship breakdown, new parent, situations at work or school – but the result is usually the same feeling of sadness, detachment and isolation from others with the idea that no-one understands.

Feelings of loneliness can be your brain's response that you need to connect with others, especially like-minded people, even though this may be the last thing you feel like doing. Have you ever felt lonely?

What was happening for you when these feelings surfaced?

What did you do or not do that you felt helped with these feelings? To combat these feelings, it is important to identify the triggers as well as what we were able to do to reduce the feeling.

Do things that make you feel good, being with others is not the only way to reduce loneliness. Finding new interests and hobbies is a great way to experience stability and connection.

If there has been a specific incident or experience that has occurred that triggered the sense of loneliness, you may feel no-one understands, but reach out to a support group as this can help provide information as well as support. Provide opportunities to share your experience that may allow you to feel heard and gain a real sense of connection, a feeling of belonging and that you are understood. This is so important, as being silenced or not expressing your feelings can also lead to loneliness.

Spend time in nature or perhaps get a pet, while this may not be an option for everyone, it has been shown to reduce loneliness and isolation.

Find like-minded people. I am part of an online book club of women that are from different parts of Ireland, we get up early twice a week and discuss the book we are reading – these can be of any description, however, the connection, relationship building and sense of belonging is not one I had anticipated, though the impact it has had on all of us is so powerful we talk about it all the time. The days we connect and have book club can be the most productive days of the week.

I encourage everyone to find what works for you and consistently make an effort. In a world where social media has many striving to be perfect, go against the grain and find your imperfect tribe, build relationships and enjoy connecting and prevent the loneliness that can impact us all.

SELF-SABOTAGE

It's something most of us do from time to time. It can be a strange one, and it comes from different places. You may be consciously or unconsciously doing it. Some of the causes range from prior relationship problems, to experiences that you've had or limiting beliefs that we've spoken about.

Self-sabotage can be the act of destroying or undermining yourself.

And while others can see how amazing we are, sometimes we self-sabotage ourselves. It's really important to recognise if you're doing this and the reasons behind it.

It can be to do with your weight. So, if you're overweight and on a diet, you may consciously sabotage your good efforts by eating the wrong foods, believing that you're always going to be in that size. Or you may be doing it unconsciously, like missing a work deadline. On the surface it seems like you're only a bit late, but actually you're afraid of failure.

You need to work out why it is you're self-sabotaging. Are you afraid of failure? Is it because of limiting beliefs, is it past experiences, is it trauma? And really be honest with yourself as to why. An example in my life is in business, I had to make a really important phone call that was going to be really good for my business and I kept procrastinating it when really it was self-sabotage because I was afraid of failure, I was afraid of the rejection. I had to work out where that came from, and I just lifted the phone then and made the call. And you know what? It all worked out. So, the story that we tell ourselves in our own minds is not always true.

And again, that is because fear of disappointing others, fear of failure, fear of success, fear of rejection or perfectionism. Self-medication for different reasons can be sabotaging your health and your wellbeing. How to stop this really is to recognise that there's something else going on.

Maybe talk to a therapist, coach or mentor. You need to be open for guidance and a safe place to understand where the self-sabotage is coming from. And call yourself out. Don't let yourself get away with it either. Once you recognise it and understand that you can overcome it, it's actually quite easy.

We all have examples of this in our lives.. And it can be limiting; it can be limiting your progress, whether it's personally or professionally. And we all deserve better.

GROWTH

Growth is so important throughout our lifetime. Staying still should never be an option. Life is for living, and we should embrace it, even the challenges.

A growth mindset is the belief that your skills and abilities are not always going to be the same.

A growth mindset will show you that intelligence can be developed, new skills can be developed. You can learn what you need to learn in order to achieve what you want to.

Growth is, despite any obstacles or challenges, you're willing to persist and overcome them.

You don't mind criticism or negative comments. You learn from them; you grow from them. You take what you need from feedback and let it go. Do not take anything personally. Part of growth, as well, I believe, are having role models in your life.

Having those people around you that help you to be inspired and their values and their ethics are what you aspire to be. Be inspired by other people's successes. Learn from them, understand what it is that got them there. I find that can be very useful.

Growth is never staying still. A growth mindset is the opposite of believing you are not good enough, that you cannot do this. A growth mindset is that you will gain the skills and knowledge that you need in order to achieve what it is that you need to achieve. Surround yourself with the right people. Use the four agreements.

Don't take anything personally. Always do your best. Be impeccable with your word. Don't make assumptions.

Learn to stand tall with your values and beliefs and know who you are and what you stand for.

Mistakes help you learn, grow and set goals to keep going. You can learn to achieve anything if you put your mind to it. You can train your brain, and there's always room for improvement. Nothing has to say stay the same way. You can grow.

Recognise that you have a choice.

Mastery takes practise, bringing growth into any situation. Put yourself in situations that are challenging. Don't give up. Keep going until you achieve what it is that you have set to achieve. A growth mindset is the belief that you can achieve it through doing what you need to do.

EMOTIONAL INTELLIGENCE

I believe that emotional intelligence is a very important skill to have. It's the ability to perceive, control and evaluate our emotions. Some research shows that emotional intelligence can be learned and strengthened, while others debate that maybe it's a characteristic you either have or you don't.

I believe the more we learn about it, the more we understand it, the more we can nurture it within ourselves. Emotional intelligence is self-awareness.

We all have different sides. It's about knowing who you are, what your personality type is, what triggers you, how you react, how you choose to respond. It is empathy that we are able to show in different situations. It's our social skills. Are you an introvert? Are you an extrovert? How do you come across? What is your favourite communication style? What motivates you? What ignites the fire within? What gets you excited?

It's about understanding what it is that you need to get motivated and self-regulation. One of the most important things that we can learn about ourselves and teach ourselves is self-motivation.

It allows us to control our emotions, understand them, know who we are, respond and not react negatively to external situations. It's our ability to control and express our emotions and how we interpret how we're feeling.

The highest level of emotional intelligence is the ability to manage our emotions effectively, regulate them, respond appropriately and understand them. This takes time. It's not necessarily something that we are taught from a young age, but it's certainly worth looking into.

It helps shape who you are. It helps you motivate yourself, learn new things. It allows you to be assertive within yourself. It allows you to choose your life path.

It allows you to be social, surround yourself with the right people, show assertiveness, create the life that you want based on the choices that you have made. There's so much more to this but you get to choose. The more you understand, the more self-aware you become. Self-management as part of your personality, social awareness and your social skills are all important factors of emotional intelligence.

PERSONALITY

There is no universal definition of what our personality is or how we come to be. It can be many different factors. It's the whole nature vs. nurture discussion. Although, I do believe our personality can change throughout our lifetime based on experiences, whether they are good or bad, and also trauma if it impacts us. Gordon Alport states personality is far too complex a thing to be thrusted in a conceptual straitjacket.

So it is all things that we are. Do you know your personality style? This is something that I have done many times over the years, especially in my career in mental health. It truly is an important thing to understand yourself, and I've mentioned it in many chapters within this book. In the early days, I would have always done the Myers Briggs[1] personality test.

It gives you a set of letters and explains a little about your personality style and maybe what's good about who you are and what you need to work on. In more recent years, I've used the Gallup[2] personality test and it appeared to capture me quite well. You answer the questions yourself as quick as you can because that's when they're honest.

---

1 mbtionline.com/?msclkid=2f483cce34661bcda7fe5f9a558d1c86
2 gallup.com/cliftonstrengths

It then gives you a detailed report on your personality type, your strengths, your weaknesses, what's a good career path to go down and why you do what you do. I already knew most of it myself, but seeing it written down really helped me to understand a little bit more about me. So, your personality, essentially, is who you are. It's a supreme realisation of why you do the things you do, why you think the way you think, why your emotions are the way they are. There are multiple sources which can provide your personality.

It can be the genetic and environmental origins that you came from, your social forces which motivates traits, behaviours and attitudes, and then also the clinical side of things. Your personality is so beautifully part of who you are. Do not ever hide it. Embrace it. Acknowledge the good, maybe the not so good.

Change what you feel you need to, but always stay true to yourself. You are unique. Understanding you and your personality is one of the most beautiful things that you can gift yourself. Write down what you like, what you don't like, what you don't understand about yourself and read about it, talk about it, listen to podcasts, get information, just learn about it. Accept who you are.

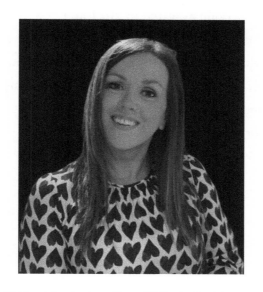

EMMA WEAVER

Emma Weaver is the founder of Mental Wealth International, an organisation supporting businesses to achieve better mental health and wellbeing within the workplace.

Emma has over twenty-three years' experience working in the mental health and wellbeing sector. Supporting adults with wellbeing, working across various sectors such as managing teams and developing services.

Founder of limitless in leadership supporting startups and entrepreneurs through an accelerator group and mentoring.

Also an international bestselling author with her debut novel, *The Blue Line*.

As an international speaker she uses her voice to champion mental wealth.

Emma is a two-time TEDx speaker, and has also curated two TEDx events in Enniskillen.

Passion Vista's one to watch in 2021 and 2021 CIO women in business leader top ten to look up to.

Ambassador for *Evolve Women, The Colours of Me* anthology, contributor to *Think Limitlessly* and partnership with many other female lead events and mental health campaigns.

Co-author of *The Wealthy Mindset.*

CONTRIBUTORS

MENTAL WEALTH
AND ME

CHET HIRANI

I didn't know what mental wealth meant or was, all the while I was going through highs and lows, and didn't know what was happening. Until something hit me.

Roughly twenty years ago (I certainly don't feel that old), I was having the time of my life. Enjoying the life of university, going out every night, coming back late and then attending lectures with minimal sleep. Also doing last-minute revision for exams. (You all know what I mean, I'm sure most of you have been there.) However, during this time, I was going through the number-one struggle I always kept to myself. That was my appearance. I associated my appearance with a lot of things – I wanted to look good for others, and I thought this would affect my chances of finding a job when I finished uni. But I never thought of looking and feeling good for myself.

I was always on the chubby side when compared to my peers, and I was called a few names along the way, which did affect me, but

I never showed this. I decided to be the centre of attention (which I still am) which made me think getting the attention was the coping mechanism.

This feeling followed me until only recently when I found the ingredients to overcome this.

After uni, I eventually found a job, which led me to spend fifteen years or more in the software tech industry. During this time, I struggled with weight issues, a divorce, alcoholism, depression, anxiety, being told I had cancer to then it not being cancer but tuberculosis, and then being told that I can never have children of my own.

The weight dropped off and I still was drinking, while getting over a divorce, but I continued to do two things. Work, because I had dreams, and teaching my martial arts class every week. Teaching the class was my only way of closing everything behind me and getting into a state of mind that made me feel fearless and in control.

I eventually got over my illness, but the alcohol was an issue, and I used not being able to have children as my excuse. I was now using this as a negative coping mechanism. I lost a lot of weight but all in a very unhealthy way. This all had to stop, and I was given an ultimatum by my now-partner.

I went to see someone, which was probably the best decision ever made. Simply because during my time speaking to them, something triggered in me. I was talking about all the good I needed to do and feel, and all the actions I needed to take for me this to happen. I had the answer to getting over this state.

This is when I understood the importance of mental wealth. In my opinion, this a combination of health and wellbeing, but it all depends on how you as a person see this, and how it can be applied and implemented into your own lives. One important factor is to be able to acknowledge the problems, and if you can't, seek support because this will be the start of better things. It was and has been for me.

This is the foundation of everything before we can move on to the next level. Take the strongest structural shape, the triangle or pyramid. Starting at the base will be the foundation, where I have learned over the years is where it all begins, and if that isn't set then moving up will be a struggle.

So, what is the foundation?

Imagine a concrete base. What are the key ingredients for this? Cement, sand, stone, water and air. Without these five ingredients, you will not make a good mix to create a solid foundation. Replacing these five ingredients with health, wellbeing, belief, consistency and acknowledgement will create your own life's cement and will create the solid foundation for your triangle to then go further.

It all starts with your overall health and wellbeing. My view on this is that if you don't get your health in order and you don't work on your wellbeing – not having the belief to visualise the change, not being consistent and not acknowledging everything around you – then you won't be in the right state of mind and you will lose focus on the direction you want to go in. That foundation needs to be rock-solid. Cracks may appear, but you'll be in a far better position to solidify this a lot quicker when you have the right mix.

I've always been an active person, involved in various types of sports, so I thought I was pretty healthy. But working out and being involved in sports is just a small part of this. I discovered that for me to start to feel good about myself I also needed to understand what was happening in the kitchen. See, 80% is what you eat and only 20% is the active side. A huge difference when having the mindset of

I've worked out so I can eat anything. I know you know what I mean, I've been there, so you're not alone. I'm associating health with my physical state. For me, this is one of the ingredients, it can vary for others. If I am not in a good physical state, then my foundation will start to crumble.

Health, to me, doesn't just mean being active, it means eating right, it means being consistent in what you need and how you want to feel. This could mean having stability in your business so that it stays healthy, improving yourself in your workplace, which will allow you to get through the hardest of times. Health also means working to be comfortable in your way of living.

Wellbeing, in my view, has no direct definition, however, the fundamental elements are having a positive emotional state and eliminating the negative states. I like to call dimensions of wellbeing to discover what works for you and how you apply it to your life, all for the better. You always want to work toward being the best version of yourself. Having the balance in place that works for you from a wellbeing perspective will allow this to take place. These dimensions can include physical, emotional, financial, social, occupational, spiritual, intellectual and environmental.

There are times when I am in an emotional state this is overshadowed by negative thoughts, and in the past, I was full of these thoughts. It felt like the world was against me and there was nothing I nor anyone could do about it. Only until I discovered what the trigger was, was I able to overcome the doubts and start to create the positive emotions within me to take over. I also went through a time when my social network was my all, only to realise they were not giving me what I wanted and needed. Instead, it was a toxic feeling, so I took drastic measures because this also affected my financial state. The measures I took were to think about who were the people I wanted to surround myself with, who were the people that will support and guide me to where I want to be. Once I discovered this, I closed off all relations with the other social network. Yes, I disconnected from them on social media, it didn't matter what they thought because I had to put myself first. I was also able to change the environment I was in, this improved dramatically, and to my surprise, I was far more alert of what I was doing and started to see results from that mindset shift instantly.

A top tip here would be to find your spiritual side. What I mean by this is take on tasks that are not directly related to your everyday life but do have an impact. For me it's martial arts – this gets me in a zone where I come out feeling better than when I entered. For you, it could be finding time to meditate. This doesn't mean just sitting down in silence and listening to the meditation. I usually take five minutes when I feel like it and just sit in silence, or read a few pages or listen to a personal development audiobook. Meditation is about focus and getting into the peak state of mind which will allow you to get through the toughest of times.

So as part of the ingredients, I have covered the top two. However, this all can only happen with the right belief and consistency in place. As they say, 'Seeing is believing.' It is the case. Visualising your aspirations and seeing them come to life has this feeling of anything is possible. You must try it. However, as much as believing is important, consistency is also key. This doesn't mean you do it for a week and everything is great. There is a reason why there needs to be consistency, it's almost like having a rhythmic flow to it. You will be in total control and eventually be the master of your own mental wealth.

The last ingredient, which tends to be the toughest of them all, is to acknowledge the issues at hand. See, the foundation can be laid with all four ingredients, but once cracks start to appear, acknowledgement is required to mend the cracks to keep things solid. Once a crack appears and you've moved to the next level – well, I will leave you to imagine what can happen. Acknowledgement doesn't have to be only what is going on around you, but also acknowledge the changes and actions of others that have a direct impact on you.

I recall a time when I was so strict on my health and wellbeing – I was at my peak. I felt great, I felt unstoppable. The belief was 100% there and I was consistent within myself. I did what I had to do. It became a habit of mine. I imagine this as being on a smooth road and if a pothole came I was able to avoid this with ease and just keep going. Until I hit a rock along the way and disjointed my path, I began to slow down. This rock was a slight shift and change in my daily routine. It meant I had to shift and be flexible in adjusting to the change. I was prepared for this, but I wasn't prepared for the unknown. I started to do things differently, still working on myself. But realised something wasn't right. Something didn't feel right. See, I acknowledge this. As soon as I feel there is something not quite right, I assess what changes are happening, why am I behaving this way. As soon as I realised what it was, I simply readjust back to what worked and how I was comfortable within myself.

So, acknowledgement is just as important as the rest. You need to reflect and go back on what has changed. As soon as the cracks start to appear, it needs to be filled as soon as you can. Now, it can take some time but the fundamental point I am making here is once you acknowledge it, you're on the right track.

To this day, I refer to myself and teach others the importance of having the right foundation set and what is required to continue and be the best version of yourself.

There is so much more meaning to health and wellbeing that has a direct impact on our lives which is why the emotional aspects play a huge part, hence the creation of mental wealth.

I am in a great place, and I ensure everyone I connect with also gets in their best state. The reminder here is to do what works for you. Once you have found your secret ingredient, don't stop going for it. Remind yourself of why you started in the first place, and it will all fall into place like a puzzle. That missing piece will be found, and once it's found, just imagine the feeling of when you complete a puzzle to feeling complete within yourself.

Remember that something I referred to at the beginning of this chapter? Well, until this day, I don't know what that something is, which is why I simply still call it 'something'.

I challenge you to go find your 'something'.

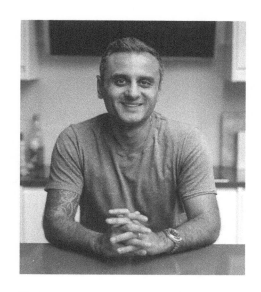

CHET HIRANI.

Chet Hirani is an international peak performance coach, speaker and podcast host. He's also a martial arts trainer that embodies the warrior spirit of humility, clarity and integrity while rigorous and extremely disciplined to bring out the best in you. He holds a Bachelor's Degree in Computer Science, a Masters in Software Engineering and has lived corporate life for fifteen years in software tech climbing up the ladder and working with executives, giving him insight into people's minds and making a better analysis of the struggles, and now enables the solution to develop people and businesses in leadership, growth and performance.

MY PERFECTIONISM BECAME MY RESPONSE TO CHILDHOOD TRAUMA

GERALDINE MC GRATH

I come from a deprived area of north-west UK. It was October 1983, I was two years old recovering from German measles. That afternoon, my mum had gone with my older sister to town to buy her very first school uniform and a record that become one of our favourite childhood songs, 'Karma Chameleon'. My lovely auntie stayed to look after me and my two sisters. During this short time, I had become very unwell. My mum arrived back home. My auntie said, 'Thank goodness you're home, Geraldine is starting to shake.' It was a prolonged febrile convulsion. My mum cried out for help, and thankfully a nurse across the road was quick to respond. The emergency services arrived and took over from here.

On arrival at the hospital, I had a severe reaction to penicillin. My mum had to wait outside the hospital room, the doctor approached and said, 'Mrs Mc Grath, did you not realise your daughter had an allergy to penicillin? You need to call Geraldine's dad to come down immediately.' I asked my mum recently how long did it feel for her waiting outside that hospital room. She said it felt like a lifetime! Several hours passed, and my mum and dad were allowed to see me, their little girl lay lifeless in the hospital cot, my face had disfigured, and I was critically ill!

Over the next two days I continued to show no signs of movement, my features were all disfigured. On day three, I opened my eyes, disorientated not knowing who my parents were, which was heartbreaking for my mum and dad. But by day six I had shown positive signs of recovery and was transferred to another hospital where I would remain for a further two weeks.

Back home were my two older sisters, three and five years old, and my newborn sister just two weeks old. Throughout the next number of weeks my parents tried their very best to visit me, but let's be realistic here, my dad had to work to provide for us and my mum was already caring for my three sisters including a two-week old baby!

In the 1980s, parents were not permitted to stay over the hospital. My dad recalls I would cry so hard when my mum had to return home, my dad stayed with me and the tears would flow once he had to leave my side.

A two-year-old little girl separated from her parents, sisters and home life. After almost three weeks in total I was then reunited with my loving family. It took six weeks for my facial features to return to my normal self.

At three years old concerns were raised about my ability to speak and the possible consequences of my illness. The youngest of our preschool class, at just three years old, I can clearly remember my speech therapist working with me regularly in the classroom environment.

The sessions were intense as my mum would also have to bring me to regular additional sessions outside of school, sitting on a big bus practising my tongue movements there and back.

Did you know that perfectionism traits often arise from psychological wounds of childhood, children who experience emotional trauma?

As a child, I constantly got told I was an old soul, mature for my age and an old head on young shoulders. I always could juggle many tasks at once. I recall at the age of eight starting our weekly grocery shop whilst my mum was seeing to my sisters in the shopping mall. I could also read the world and everyone around me, measuring it for perceived danger and adapting my behaviour to suit the environment. Was it a superpower? It was a very clever coping strategy for dealing with my childhood trauma.

My parents both had significant trauma in their early childhoods and throughout life. With mental health difficulties in both families, throughout life there were times where this left them being incredibly emotional.

So, throughout my childhood, I became the best at everything I could.

I recall having a very happy-go-lucky, carefree childhood in Manchester where I was born. My parents were both Irish and they had the vision to bring us up in their home country. This happened in 1992 and we left Manchester for a new chapter in County Fermanagh when I was ten years old.

The initial excitement of our move to Ireland felt like a holiday. Having one term to finish in primary school, little did I know the happy-go-lucky, carefree Geraldine would slowly become lonely and isolated.

Did I have the courage to be imperfect?

Pushed by fear from bullying, my vulnerability was clear to be seen. For the first time in my life, my imperfections were being called out by the bullies. My appearance, my weight and my English accent, to name a few. I was grateful to have the support of my good new friends, however, I can still recall the hurt, sadness and emptiness within.

So, let's look at what triggers perfectionism: fear of disapproval, insecurity, anxiety and insecure early attachment in childhood can all result in perfectionism.

Over the next two years, my battle to avoid the bullying started early in the mornings, crying to Mum to keep me at home with her. This would continue in the car until the school bus arrived, some days I went on to school, on the tough days I returned home with Mum.

The traits of perfectionism were becoming my new normal! Loneliness, isolation, pushed by fear, low confidence, low self-esteem, an all-or-nothing approach, fixing things, people-pleasing, highly critical and so hard on myself.

Yet another imperfection resurfaces, the ability of my speech. Did I have the courage to be imperfect?

I would sit with my hands sweating under the table in fear of being asked to read out loud, what if I stuttered my words? What if I couldn't pronounce a word? This bubbly ten-year-old was soon to have low confidence and self-esteem.

You see, the root of perfectionism is believing your self-worth is based on your achievements!

Reflecting, I always wondered why it took me so much longer to complete my work. It had to be to a certain standard, it had to be as perfect as I could get it! For sure, this was an area where I became highly critical and hard on myself with an all-or-nothing approach.

The fear was so real! I didn't dare to be imperfect. I recall in secondary school avoiding the corridors, arriving at class earlier or leaving class later where I believed the bullying would happen, I would hear it begin before I even started walking up the corridor. I would pass one group of bullies to go to the staircase, before I reached the top of those stairs the next chants would be heard.

For so many years I questioned myself, *Why me?* I didn't speak back to them, I tried to fit in – only now I realise they identified that vulnerability within me, so I was their easy target!

According to Dr Robin Alter, there are three reasons why children bully.

1. Because they were bullied, and they are giving another what they got from someone else.
2. Because they think by putting someone else down, they will put themselves up.
3. Because someone is different from them, and they are threatened when someone is different.

If only I had understood this at a much earlier stage in my life! Let's think about this, as a perfectionist I was doing to myself what the other children had done to me.

As Brené Brown quotes, perfectionism is a twenty-ton shield that we lug around thinking it will protect us when, in fact, it's the thing that's preventing us from being seen and taking flight!

My way of feeling adequate and in control of my world was perfection.

Any failure on my part not only made me feel like I didn't deserve to be alive but like I had brought anything bad that ever happened to me upon myself for not being good enough. As I got older, this perfectionism converted into people-pleasing, constant apologising for everything even if I didn't do anything but breathe. Some bumped into me in the street, I apologised for it, seeking constant validation for things, looking to others to make decisions, and the inability to truly absorb compliments without feeling like an imposter.

THE SHIFT IN MY LIFE

What was the shift, that turning point in my life?

At thitry-five years of age in 2016 at a business convention, I had my first introduction to personal development and growth. That day, I listened to several speakers, and the seed was planted. Light bulbs started to shine with endless possibilities available to me. It felt like I had been living under a rock for most of my life. The only form of personal development I had completed was counselling. Throughout the coming years, I became hungry to learn, attending numerous trainings, conferences, events and workshops to constantly upskill. I started to see life through a broader lens. If I could describe this to you, visualise a large egg. Initially, it was hairlines that appeared, however, within me I still was feeling very stuck.

A loving busy mum of four, and wife, I was spinning lots of plates. Life will bring you challenges that you must adapt to and add to that already busy schedule.

However, certain personal challenges in 2019/2020 led me to a life coach/counsellor. I spent many, many sessions with him, we worked together for almost a year. On one of these calls, towards the end of the session, my life coach softly mentioned for me to look up the traits of perfectionism and do a little research. I looked it up online, but I didn't fully connect with it as my self-awareness wasn't there yet.

Throughout my journey of personal development, I worked so hard and committed to learning new practices. However, the patterns continued of being my worst critic. Self-doubt, self-sabotage, procrastinating, negative self-talk and overthinking – the list goes on of my behaviours and habits.

The ongoing struggles I identified were:

- People-pleasing – The need to please others at my own expense. I agreed to keep others happy even though it wasn't sitting with my gut, it would scream at me. I still would continue to smile and agree.
- Boundaries – I still had work to complete with my boundaries, creating boundaries that would keep me safe and healthy. Creating healthy boundaries would enable me to keep aligned moving forward on my journey.
- Indecisive – Looking for the approval of others to make decisions that I could have made myself, however, I lacked the confidence.
- The peacekeeper – pushing difficult situations under the mat so that I didn't have to face them head-on.

I now have realised that I've been hanging on to this coping strategy for dear life because it's the one that has made me feel the safest for so long. But if I'm being honest, 2021 was a very impolite awakening in terms of disrupting the effectiveness of this coping strategy. I didn't feel safe, I didn't feel in control, I didn't feel creative or appreciated, I didn't feel perfect. I felt flawed and I felt human, and I was uncomfortable in my skin and head.

What did my world look like from the outside in? I achieved

huge success throughout this time in my business. I reached levels I never believed were possible for me, however, on the inside I was still hurting.

In early 2021 I was offered the opportunity to complete my very first TEDx Talk.

When I started to create my talk the word perfectionism appeared so many times on my screen, the brightest light bulb went on, that moment it clicked! At forty years of age, the jigsaw pieces started to connect.

I revisited the traits of perfectionism, and the connection to it was so real! All the traits, patterns and behaviours were so familiar.

Almost five years into my journey of personal development I had an awakening of self-awareness. I took time to evaluate where I was on my journey of personal development and growth.

I continued to create deeper levels of self-awareness within me. You see, self-awareness is so important, when we have a better understanding of ourselves, we can experience ourselves as unique and separate individuals.

As Tony Robbins quotes, 'Self-awareness is one of the rarest of human commodities. I don't mean self-consciousness where you're limiting and evaluating yourself. I mean being aware of your patterns.'

In January 2021, I chose a word that would represent the year for me. That word is authenticity, to be true to me and who I am. On 5 August 2021, the courage for me to be imperfect was born! I delivered my TEDx Talk – *Do You Have the Courage to Be Imperfect?*

My TEDx Talk emphasises the word 'imperfect'.

Imperfect spells *I'm perfect* because everyone is perfect in their imperfect ways. My message and significance of imperfect for you is:

- Inspiration – Have the inspiration within you to discover yourself.

Discover your creativeness within.

- Meaningful – To live a meaningful life of being your true authentic self.
- Peace – To find your inner peace within you to focus on your natural energy of joy.
- Empathy – Express empathy to understand and share the feelings of another.
- Reconciliation – To accept or come to terms with something you must deal with.
- Fabulous – Remind yourself each day that you are fabulous.
- Expressive – Empower your ability to be expressive and open.
- Captain – To take control of your life you are the captain of your ship.
- Thankful – To practice gratitude for you and your life.

Following my TEDx Talk, it brought a lot to the surface for me. I revisited my counsellor from earlier years I had attended at certain times of challenges in my adult life. I honestly felt I couldn't try any harder, even though I had made significant progress I still felt something was missing. She identified that it was my time to reflect, time to slow down, time to ground myself and open myself up more for opportunities. As she knows all too well my fondness for taking responsibility for everyone and everything and for beating myself up for failing at anything.

Moving forward, I identified that I had to explore self-development further and take a deep dive within myself. I needed to figure out how to let go of this perfectionism and learn to be okay with being human. I've had to let go of any idea that I can protect myself from trauma or harm because none of us can. Bad things can and will happen. But they aren't a reflection of our worth and they do not make us any less deserving of love. I'm going to hold onto that piece of the healing journey and slowly let it sink in, flaws and all.

From here my soul-searching journey began. I am so proud of how far I have come on this journey. Today, I am still on this journey progressing each day; it will always be a journey of learning and self-development to become a better person than I was yesterday.

Difficult roads lead to beautiful destinations. I'm a woman who has pushed deep within herself, went to the darkest of places to discover her true purpose in life. I see my journey as a bamboo tree. It took several years of working on my roots before I could show up as Geraldine Mc Grath – the unstoppable mentor. My word for 2022 is 'radiate' to radiate my warm gift of energy to empower many women to become the unstoppable version of themselves.

A fierce advocate for women to break habits and behaviours holding them back by helping them see the fuel and power in self-awareness, reconnection and having tools to beat self-sabotage and become the most unstoppable version of themselves.

Let me bring you back to the very start, that day in October 1983, the day when my beautiful mum bought the record 'Karma Chameleon' – the song that represents that happy-go-lucky young girl's childhood!

Its meaning represents equality – as the lyrics go, 'Loving would be easy if your colours were like my dreams, red, gold and green.' The red represents the blood of all living things in the world, the gold is for all the treasures in the world that people cherish and the green is for the earth that people walk on.

The song is about the terrible fear of alienation that people have, the fear of standing up for the one thing you believe in.

My wish for you is that my message will give you the strength and hope that you too can overcome the traits of a perfectionist and become your true authentic self.

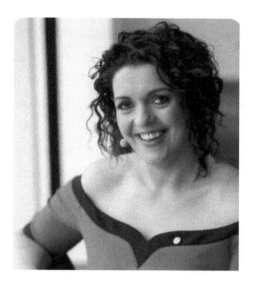

GERALDINE MC GRATH

I am unstoppable.

Geraldine is a fierce advocate for helping women break habits and behaviours that hold them back, and to help them discover their unique gifts and passions through the raw fuel of self-awareness. Her goal is to empower women to share their gifts and light with others to make a positive impact throughout the world.

Geraldine is dedicated to helping women overcome obstacles and reach their full potential through self-discovery and personal empowerment. Specialising in one-to-one 'Intuitive Mentorship' and 'The Unstoppable Evolution' – A group program alongside further 'Unstoppable Offerings'.

She is the host of *Radiate Realness* podcast, creating real and raw conversations by sharing the beautiful gift of vulnerability to empower others.

A speaker, a TEDx Speaker, *Do You Have the Courage to be Imperfectly Perfect* and communication lead for TEDx Enniskillen.

Geraldine is also an experienced mentor and facilitator, focusing on 'Intuitive Mentorship', facilitating to use her voice and gift of connection to create conversations and awareness around suicide prevention.

A suicide first aid tutor, city and guilds recognised and an addictions trainer and facilitator. In 2023 it's a reflection of sorrow that our death by suicide rates continue to increase. It's time to break the silence, to break down the stigma and create important conversations. It's time to save lives!

WRITE FROM THE HEART

Rosie Keaney

The darkness it felt so heavy, it was 28 August 2018 and I had closed the doors to my business overnight. My life had changed forever that day, all I had ever known over the past fifteen years had fallen apart in a moment's breath.

At the time I was eight months pregnant with my long and much anticipated fourth child, what was to be an exciting new chapter in my life, so I had thought had been stolen from me, the pages torn out of my book, my plans, dreams and visions destroyed, blew up in smoke, it felt like the pages of my life had been swept away.

The days and weeks ahead were long and weary, I woke up each day feeling lost, numb, like I was a stranger in my own body, everything was different and I felt empty. I just wanted my old life back, the familiar day-to-day routine, even if I was a little bit unhappy in that world – if the truth be told it was the security and familiarity I missed the most.

I did not recognise the person I was becoming, so swallowed up by fear and guilt it was eating me alive. This had been building up over several years. I was a shadow of my former self, the woman who once stood before me was a confident and self-assured businesswoman, but now I was an anxious and nervous mum of four.

I remember the day I had returned to the business premises to remove my belongings and allow others to collect theirs. I brought my four-week-old newborn baby with me, my sister Dean and my husband Nick there as always to support me, I would be lost without them, they never left my side.

That day when I walked into the nursery, the building felt alien to me, there was no familiar sound of children's voices and laughter, just a deadly silence. There was no heating on since we had last occupied the building and as it was the midst of winter, I felt a cold chill upon entering – both spiritually and physically it felt dead to me, like this part of my life no longer existed.

No more were the warm and happy faces, the bright walls with artwork had gone, the colour had drained from the walls right before my very own eyes. Holding my baby so closely and hiding myself away in the baby room where I could feed my newborn baby to avoid any contact with familiar faces for fear of retribution.

The days and weeks ahead were a blur. I had taken myself off social media for the cruel comments were all too much for me to handle, the kind comments were much valued as they allowed me to feel love, but there was no running away from the harsh and cruel words. Funnily enough though no-one could hate me more than I hated myself right then.

I was thankful for the time at home with my newborn baby, I did not want to ever leave the house. The thought of having to drive into my local town filled me with so much fear and anxiety I could not bring myself to face anyone.

Looking back now I was trapped in a vortex of shame and guilt, I felt numb to almost every emotion. I was just getting through each day. When I was at home I felt safety surrounded by those familiar walls. What I didn't recognise at the time was I had entered a depressive state of mind. I class myself as one of the lucky ones as my family showed me love and kindness like no other, and their love helped to heal me.

The first step for me was when I was gently guided by my sister Dean to go to a mother-and-baby group, the day arrived and I was almost ready to make an excuse to not go, I was so used to doing this, as it was easier for my anxiety to stay at home in my natural surroundings.

This particular day things were different, I felt like I could do this. I went to the church with my baby to say a few prayers for some Dutch courage and walked in the direction of the baby group. I was greeted outside the church by two familiar faces (my sister and cousin) who were there for moral support and to make sure I was going in the right direction, of course.

After attending the group, I felt happy within myself this was the first big step for me, I felt welcomed and valued within the group and not judged. I was beginning to realise that by facing my fears it was going to only make me stronger and I needed to push myself out of my comfort zone this was a very important part of my journey.

This was the beginning of my self-healing journey. Step by step, day by day I started to leave the house more. Even though I felt anxious and fearful, I needed to push myself as it was up to me to put the work in now – no-one else could do this for me.

I had become a tropic ambassador in January 2019. This business talked to my soul, I loved everything about it – the people, the company ethics, the leadership, the passion – it was like a dream come true. This business reminded me of all the goodness in the world. I was connecting with many beautiful souls who had also experienced trauma is some shape or form and had found tropic too in their times of desperation. I was discovering we all have our own difficulties and challenges to face in life. Tropic had reignited a spark within me, it reminded me of my beautiful gift of how I used to see the beauty in everyone and everything.

I started to read again, my first book was *Quiet* by Fearn Cotton, I was so relieved to be able to relate to the book and the negative self-talk at the time I had been unaware it had been so bad. My subconscious was very aware of it. I couldn't bring myself to write down my thoughts and feelings as I was finding it so much easier to supress them. Although it had opened my mind a little, this was the start of my awareness of my thinking process, my awakening.

I needed to go through a process of self-love. When I started to look for another job, I felt the same feelings of unworthiness I felt after closing my business. I didn't deserve a second chance at employment, who would want to employ me? I eventually got my first job in Next, which was a completely different environment to what I was used to, I was so pleased and grateful for the job I embraced the new opportunity.

Within three weeks of starting my new job in Next, I received two other job offers from interviews I had attended. One of them was with a leading parenting charity and the other was a part-time lecturer in my local college – both dream jobs. This was a huge boost to my shattered confidence. Things were starting to look up, perhaps I could work again in a job I loved and deserve happiness again. Within the next couple of weeks, I was unable to start my new position as COVID-19 had hit and we were told to work from home.

During COVID-19 I had never been so happy to see face masks, if only they had been around during my own pandemic. Spending time at home was a blessing for me, I had feelings of anxiety, fear of the unknown, fear for my family. Like everyone else in the country, although this felt like familiar territory for me. I had been here before, these feelings of despair were not unfamiliar to me. I discovered that by writing and sharing my thoughts I was able to help others who were feeling the same.

There was a time when I thought I would never be able to face my fears again, but through self-healing I have came to realise we are all the same, we all feel fear when doing something new, even those that don't show fear feel fear. I had closed many doors because I had felt unworthy, but this was all about to change.

Every day I was getting stronger, I was still writing posts and sharing them on my social media. Writing is my absolute passion; it always has been my happy place. I had just been too distracted to notice in the past. When I started working for Parenting NI I felt so welcome and valued by my new manager Maria, and the team to this day, she and they have no idea how much they helped and supported me at that time.

For the right people you are not too sensitive, too emotional, too whatever else other people's opinions may be of you, find your tribe and they will love you for exactly who you are.

Fast-forward almost three years and I am overwhelmed with my progression. I have organised Christmas markets in my local community which had terrified me half to death at the time, as that would mean facing the very people who I had let down, but I am so proud of myself for putting myself out there, opportunities were arising and I was able to allow myself to go for them.

In December 2021, I had entered to take part in TEDx Enniskillen, my first ever TEDx talk, in my local community and this was a breakthrough moment for me. I had so many learnings about myself and my healing journey. I made some amazing lifelong connections and friendships.

In 2022 I set up my own business Dream Big Events fulfilling my purpose and passion in business, and I had the opportunity to organise my first event for an international keynote speaker from Australia.

There will be times your experiences will return to remind you of your fears, we need to remember that by facing our fears, we are becoming a more powerful version of ourselves.

Having faith got me through my difficult time:

FAITH
F IS FOR FAMILY

Family is my safe place. This is the place for me where people wanted to still love me, you will feel very much unloved and lonely in times of difficulty, so you need to take that love in. Try not to block them out beacuse they are looking to help you.

Whenever I talk of family, I am not just talking about your partner, children, siblings, I am talking about those people in the community that believe in you and want to help you.

Those closest to you will have your best interests at heart and will offer you much support and guidance on your journey. It is so important that you begin to trust others.

They will encourage you to remember all those parts of you that you had forgotten. They want you back.

Think of all the people who have supported you throughout your life, each and every family or friend has the skills to help you move forward. Also think about the best person who will be honest and give you the advice you need.

A IS FOR ACTION

When I hit rock bottom, I didn't know what I was good at anymore, I didn't know what I could do or what I even wanted to do. I had lost me. When you hit rock bottom it is a dark and lonely place; there are no road maps, no directions, no sat nav's, you need to be there alone with your thoughts.

First of all, acknowledge your feelings, listen to your innermost feelings, it's okay to cry, it's okay to be regretful, it's okay to be sad, if you feel ashamed, feel ashamed we need to breathe through those feelings, try not to push them aside, you need to allow these feelings to flow to heal.

Fear disappears the moment you take action.

If you feel stuck in your life it means you need to change something, you all need exploration and growth. The only way to make change happen and get what you want is by pushing yourself, push yourself to get out of bed and not to press snooze, push yourself to meet new people, push yourself to take the class.

Don't wait for the day for you to feel motivation to do something, don't wait for the perfect moment, don't wait, you will waste days, weeks, months of your life if you keep waiting, what are you waiting for?!

Your fears will create many barriers in your head and will stop you from doing what you want to do. It is so important to step outside of your comfort zone. Start to get comfortable with being uncomfortable.

I IS FOR INTUITION

We all know that gut feeling when an alarm bell goes off – that's our inner guidance and we need to listen to our intuition what is your gut telling you.

Your intuition can be drowned out by the opinions of others, trust your gut, do not worry if others don't quite see things as you do, we are all different otherwise the world would be a very boring place.

Believe in your intuition, sometimes I was guided to do certain things which involved me putting myself out there again, I used to hear the voices in my head, *Are you crazy!* But I knew this is what I had to do. I am so glad I did.

By following your intuition, you will see new opportunities and have the chance to build new skills and new talents, ones you never thought possible if you just keep pushing yourself into the unknown.

Remember you have your own talents, dreams and visions, believe that you can your passion can be reignited. Bring back your spark!

T IS FOR TEACH
STUDY, PRACTICE AND TEACH

Anything you are passionate about go take that course, the seminar, read the book about it, engross yourself into that subject and build your knowledge around that.

If you are convincing yourself you are fine about not having that dream business, not having that perfect relationship, not having that healthy lifestyle, stop, you can have everything you want by pushing yourself and working hard.

Find your passion again – this enabled me to feel whole again, what is yours?

Is it creating art, playing music, dance , singing, find what lights you up.

I am a creative writer, I am known for my dreamlike qualities, find that passion that you get lost in and time stands still for you, you can forget everything in that moment.

Divert all your energies to that passion as eventually that feel-good factor will tip the scale against that very hard time in your life, you will begin to feel more positive when you move towards your natural talent and feel more like you.

Teach others what you have learned and become a beacon of hope by sharing your experiences. We are not alone on this path, we all need to stand together.

Your energy and vibration will start to rise when you start to talk about your passion and not your misfortune.

H IS FOR HEALING

You need to take time to reflect on your situation; it is important to do the work on yourself whether that is through, meditation, journaling, self-care, spending time with family and friends, whatever that looks like for you.

My motivational speaking journey has provided me with a life-changing opportunity to work on myself, I thought I was healed but I have come to realise that healing is lifelong, we need to do the work. By helping others I am healing too.

You can train your brain to see life more positively by having a mindset of gratitude this can help to improve your life.

FINALLY, THE IMPORTANCE OF SELF-FORGIVENESS

In the words of Trent Shelton, 'We all have dreams that have failed in our lives; it takes losing everything to make you realise you can gain better things.'

For a number of years, I had not forgiven myself, I was so hard because I had lost who I was, I was unrecognisable to myself, I have learnt that these difficult experiences are invaluable life lessons for growth, I have no regrets.

I have learnt that through having faith in me, my family supported me to be strong.

I took action to change my life.

I can hear my intuition more clearly.

I can teach and help others through my life experience.

I can heal through acceptance and self-healing practices.

You are free to do what you want to do you.

***

So my message to you today is when we move forward from difficulty we need to let go of the hurt and move on with our lives. Don't carry that shame or regret with you. You will waste years of your life. Let go and start the next chapter, allow yourself second chances because we all deserve them.

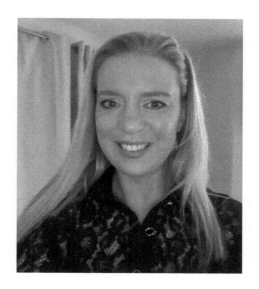

ROSIE KEANEY

Hi everyone, my name is Rosie Keaney, and I am a proud mum of four and wife to one. I am the founder of my new business Dream Big Events. I have always been a dreamer; like the business name, I love to dream big, I happily live in my imagination and love to dream and visualise new ideas, visions and projects.

Dream Big Events is all about creating opportunities for businesses, charities and non-profit organisations. As a visionary, strategist, planner and creator, I can bring your dream event to reality, making and creating an extraordinary event.

I have been in business for almost twenty years. I am passionate about business and thoroughly enjoyed studying my BSC in business studies alongside running my family business. I was in the fortunate position to apply in practise what I was learning in theory, and it changed my thought process completely. My four younger sisters, mum and dad and I had established two day nurseries and a children's indoor play centre in Enniskillen over the past fifteen years, so there was lots of learning in business development each and every day.

In December 2021 I had enrolled for my first TEDx Talk in Enniskillen which was held in the Ardhowen in June this year. It was the most profound experience of my life – other than my children and husband, of course. I healed as a direct result of this process as I was able to revisit some of the feelings I had bottled up and let them go.

TEDx helped me to remember my promise to myself after I closed my business, I promised I wanted to help others going through a difficult time in their life after what I had been through. This is my purpose and a big part of my future. I intend to do motivational talks and help others through my own personal business and life journey, and Dream Big Events is very much a part of that too.

WHAT'S THE POINT OF TALKING TO PEOPLE, ANYWAY?

Sinead Welsh

We've all been there. We've all felt stressed and worried about something, probably even on a daily or weekly basis. But what have you done with those stresses and worries? Have you unloaded them with the age-old belief that a problem shared is a problem halved? Have you figured out how to manage them to bring your calm and balance back? Or have you had those debilitating thoughts in your head that end up leading to procrastination, self-doubt and a rabbit hole of spiralling negative emotions and toxic thoughts?

I can't tell you! I can't tell anyone! I don't want to bother them! No-one will ever believe me! Maybe it will just go away?! These are some of the thoughts we have that can lead to barriers preventing us from talking to someone right when we need it most, and this can lead to a tidal wave of new problems. Many of us want to take that step to talk to someone to share our worries, but stigma, embarrassment and sometimes even shame can freeze us in our tracks.

I'd like to tell you about Rian.

RIAN'S STORY:

At age twenty-one, a student at university living with two other young men, Rian was proud that he lived a great life. They partied hard, as he said most students do, they laughed often, and Rian even managed to attend most of his lectures and pass his first two years of study.

Anyone looking objectively would have observed Rian as a tall, confident, very vocal and successful young man, because that's how he wanted to be seen and thought of by his peers, academics and family.

Two years later, now aged twenty-three, Rian visited me in my office as part of some qualitative in-house research I was undertaking. I hold a professional interest in seeking to understand the power of speaking out instead of suffering in silence.

Rian sat on my black leather seat with a warm mug of coffee in hand and started to tell me about his actual truth of never wanting to talk to anyone about how he was feeling back then at university.

I can tell you that Rian's real story was far from the perfect picture that he had portrayed so convincingly for so long.

On the outside, for example, what you see is Rian dancing, you see him drinking, you see him partying, you see him hugging and you see him kissing and smiling and having such great fun.

But that's what you see. That's what Rian wants you to see.

Behind closed doors there was a sense of sadness, a sense of loneliness, a sense of failure, stigma and guilt ... which created a paralysing fear of speaking out at all.

When Rian sat in my office looking eye to eye at me, it was clear

– 'uni Rian' was not the real Rian at all.

Rian was wearing a mask. I'm sure you've heard this metaphor before. We wear masks to protect ourselves, our vulnerable selves, our inner true selves. We don't want to stand out, we don't want people to see what we perceive as weaknesses or faults or failures and so we project a version of ourselves that we think is acceptable and popular. We have a desire and a need to fit in and be liked, and this is nowhere more evident than on the social media platforms that people use on a daily basis.

What's your social media mask – what persona do you want people to see of you? It's so common to see people posting beautiful photographs of endlessly happy moments, of successes and achievements, of well-mannered children, of beautiful clothes in beautifully toned and tanned bodies, huge smiles, luxurious holidays and loving relationships. But are they happy underneath it all? Is it the truth? We all get a kick out of the likes, the shares and the lovely positive comments. And that's okay, but are these masks and personas hiding something else? Are they making you feel worse about yourself because you know that it isn't how you're feeling inside? Are these posts of you wearing your mask stopping friends and family realising that you are struggling and that you need to talk? Are they stopping us in our tracks, stopping us from talking because we don't want to break the illusion of our happy, carefree life?

Are they doing more harm than good if we are not asking for support when we need it?

Back on my office black leather seat, Rian was grasping his coffee cup tight, wrapping both hands around it when he was brave, open and honest with me. He was confident and capable to talk, while I listened to his true story about the drinking and gambling.

The drinking started with that one cool refreshing pint at the bar and quickly escalated to drinking the next and the next day as well. Eventually this lead to the alcohol-fuelled fights and depressive hangovers. Then gambling also became a part of Rian's world. Initially, it was just for fun. It started with a £5 bet on a Saturday, spiralling quickly out of control to a bet on every single horse running that day. He could now place his bets online so no-one would ever have to find out, because Rian didn't want them to.

In many cases, families don't even know that there are problems or addictions because the victims find a way to mask it so well. They choose unhealthy ways to manage their pains and stressors and then this escalates to regular escapism, reliance and addiction. And so, they find a way to hide their hurts and their worries and unhelpful and harmful habits because they have reached a stage where they can't manage without their 'coping' mechanism and their crutch. These victims often become masters at hiding and manipulating, and this can lead to devastating effects for the victim and their close family and friends. We've heard it all too often about the heartbroken family and friends saying, 'I didn't even know he was addicted until he was gone.'

Rian continued to speak openly about the fake mask he wore so well. He told me about the night he fell to his knees on the floor, alone in his dark, cold university bedroom and broke down crying. And he knew that he just had to get out of there, he couldn't avoid these feelings any longer.

Rian didn't want to die, but he didn't want to go on the way things were either. So, he left university that night and made the long journey home.

Have you ever reached a low point in your life?

Perhaps you have reached for that chocolate or ice cream. Perhaps you have reached for that bottle of wine or bottle of whisky. Maybe it is the cannabis or lines of cocaine?

You know, a lot of things we do in life are to try to make ourselves feel better. We want to escape the pain we are feeling, and that is how many people fall into the trap of using unhealthy and even dangerous coping mechanisms, which can lead to much bigger problems.

But can you imagine if we, and those we love, reached out to talk to someone much earlier on, instead of reaching for those unhealthy and even dangerous ways to escape or cope?

WHAT WAS THE POINT TALKING TO ME THAT DAY, ANYWAY?

Rian stated that he felt a sense of release – in his own words, 'It felt almost therapeutic to get it all out.' We were recording Rian's story with the hope that by sharing it, maybe, just maybe it could help and encourage one other uni student who was alone and sad in their cold university bedroom. We are using Rian's story and so many more like it as a beacon of hope for others.

Rian was speaking the truth, and the truth always resonates!

So, what exactly helped Rian? Rian was able to talk to his mother and then his father.

WHAT WAS THE POINT IN TALKING TO HIS PARENTS, ANYWAY?

Well, for Rian, they listened to him, they believed him, they did not judge him and they did not tell him what to do next. Those initial conversations were so powerful. This was the turning point for Rian.

Unfortunately, we do know that this is not everyone's experience, not everyone can speak to their parents. But is there another adult in their life that they trust, is there another adult in their life that they know that they can turn to? Perhaps an extended family member, teacher, a lecturer or a neighbour? Having an adult in our life who believes in us, who supports us and who we know we can be open and honest with is so important. None of us want to be judged, none of us want to feel that someone disapproves of us or doesn't believe us.

Next, instead of texting his friends, Rian met them face to face. When he talked to them, it became apparent that they had no clue whatsoever how Rian had been feeling for so long, and Rian was right: unless you talk about it, how can anyone know?

WHAT'S THE POINT IN TALKING TO YOUR FRIENDS, ANYWAY?

By being brave and talking to people you trust, feeling that vulnerability but doing it anyway, this can be the first powerful step towards improved mental health and feeling connected. The first step to processing and untangling worried thoughts. Seeking help from loved ones, trusted adults or professionals is not weak – it is the way to win! It is the way to get troubling thoughts and worries out of our head – even saying them out loud can help ease the burden on our minds.

Let's go even further: could telling our real-life stories help others to see the light?

Experts call it 'see-feel-change'. This is an approach that fuels action by sparking emotion and using the power of storytelling and peer-to-peer connections to create powerful, heartfelt associations.

Would you believe it if I told you that the compelling element of telling real-life stories, according to my work, is the brilliant fact that they are NOT perfect! Actually, they are less structured, less polished and less formal – which in turn is more attractive and engaging for the listener because they can connect at an authentic level.

Telling and observing stories of others can offer a glimmer of hope. Stories can raise awareness of stressors in mental health, and real-life stories can reduce stigma. Stories allow us to feel a sense of connection to others and they can help us get ideas to make simple daily positive changes for ourselves, if we want to change. Think about it, do you feel better knowing that you're not the only one facing challenges? Do you feel better knowing that other people have bad days too and that other people don't have it all figured out just yet either? Do you feel better knowing that you don't have to have the 'perfect' social media life to have a good life? When we know that someone else has gone through something similar to us and figured out how to cope and how to live a good life, then it gives us hope for ourselves, hope for our future and the hope that we can learn how to cope and live a good life as well.

Do you have a story to share? Every single one of us do, and I'd like tell you about how – as an experienced mental health advocate and social work specialist – I got something so wrong.

In difficult times or times of crisis many of us jump instantly to thinking that we have the power to fix people, the power to save someone, that we have the answers and solutions they need. But we need to learn that we don't have that power, nor is it our job to fix anyone else, we can only work on ourselves!

I'm learning that all I really need to do is be there and listen. There is power in zero words!

It was a gorgeous Saturday. I had had a great week and I was off out for dinner to my favourite Indian restaurant with my friends. I was in a super good mood. I'm in the car singing my favourite Meghan Trainor song ... when it all changed. I went from being genuinely happy to a state of complete shock, sadness and confusion.

You see, I had received a call from my friend's husband, Jack. Jack was a solid 6ft tall, dark-haired confident man, and he phoned me sobbing profusely. I could hardly make out a word he was saying! In-between the irregularly fast breaths, he told me how my best friend Jill had attempted to end her own life!

Is she dead? Is she in hospital? What about the kids? These thoughts were frantically going around my head and my heart rate was through the roof.

BUT thank goodness, for now, Jill was safe and alive wanting to remain at home with Jack and the kids. They had a safety plan and agreement that Jill would not hurt herself overnight, but she wanted to see ME first thing in the morning.

My mind, as usual, instantly jumped to how can I fix Jill! But I should not try to fix Jill, because I can NOT fix others. I can only work on me.

We know that the majority of people who feel suicidal do not actually want to die; they do not want to live the life they have, and they just want their PAIN to end. They want to escape their pain.

This distinction may seem small, but it is very important. I learned this from the Samaritans literature.

WHAT'S THE POINT TALKING TO PROFESSIONALS, ANYWAY?

It is really important to remember that the people in charities like the Samaritans are trained professionals who are waiting to listen to you and they are hard to shock. They are compassionate and kind and there is nothing you can tell them that they haven't already heard before. When you call them, they are not there to judge you and everything you tell them is confidential. They will listen to you, and they will believe you. These professionals don't want to tell you what to do, they want you to decide what steps you would like to take and they want you to choose what's best for you.

But it's also important to remember that we are all different, we have different personalities, interests, values and beliefs, so this could mean that the first person you talk to may not be the right fit for you! This can be extremely disheartening and frustrating for someone who has worked up the courage to make that call and had to muster the courage to find their voice. But that doesn't mean there is no hope. It might mean you have to make that effort and find that courage again so that you can find the right person for you to talk to – but they are out there!

It's now the morning after the dreaded call and I'm on my way to Jill's house.

I take a deep breath and I get out of the car. It was so cold and the rain was pouring down. I slowly walked across the concrete yard, with my heart racing because I didn't know what I was walking in to. I knocked on the front door and Jill slowly opened it.

I'll always remember Jill's pink nightgown, tied at the waist; I'll always remember her matching hot pink fluffy bedroom slippers. But I will never forget her face. Jill's eyes told me that she was in a serious state of despair. With a sad look on my face too, tears in my eyes, lump in my throat, trying to keep my head held high for Jill, I opened out my arms as wide as I could. And Jill hugged me, one of the tightest embraces of our lives, and I whispered into her ear, 'I love you.'

There was lots of tea and lots of tears, and I focused on applying the best advice I had, from adapting my favourite poem by Ralph Roughton MD *On Listening*. Just be there and just listen and let there be silences.

Jill is not helpless – yes, maybe discouraged and sad, but not helpless.

Listen to her.

Do not talk and do not judge her – just be there and just hear her.

For when you do something for Jill that she can do for herself, you contribute to her fear and inadequacy.

But when you accept as a simple fact that she feels how she feels, no matter how irrational, then Jill can quit trying to convince you and get about the business of understanding what's behind this irrational feeling.

And when that's clear, the answers are obvious to Jill, and she does not need advice.

So please do not try to fix Jill, just hear her and if you want to talk, wait ... and then Jill will listen to you.

So to conclude ... what's the point talking to people, anyway? ... The response you get might just shock you as most people genuinely care. If you are listened to, believed and offered space to make your own decisions, this can liberate you to regain control. The simple act of saying things out loud to someone can also help you to feel better sooner rather than later. Getting things out of your head can help you to work out how you are thinking and feeling about different situations and it can help you begin to understand the impact it is having on you. More importantly, it can start you on the journey to work out what the next steps to managing, coping or figuring things out are – for you.

And the one thing I relearned from my childhood during my research was by BT – it's good to talk.

What's your story and who could benefit from you sharing it?

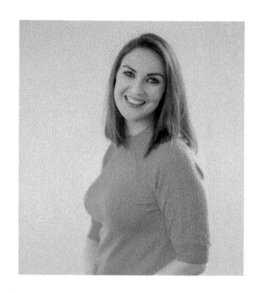

SINEAD WELSH

I am trained in social work from Queen's University Belfast, a mother of three wonderful young children. In 2007 I moved to Melbourne and lived there for ten years working for the Australian Government as a child protection manager, case conference chair lady, court officer, family law court liaison advisor and professional trainer. I held the child and adolescent mental health portfolios. I worked alongside Victoria Police around the establishment of the child sexual assault and family violence investigation teams.

HOW DECLUTTERING YOUR HOME IMPROVES YOUR WELLBEING

Sharon Mc Nulty

EMOTIONAL

As a professional home and business organiser, I organise and transform my clients' homes and I see firsthand how the space we live and work in significantly impacts our mood, productivity and mental wellbeing. It's hard to feel relaxed in a messy home, and many of my clients report they feel anxious and overwhelmed by the mess, but they just don't know where to start. They are continually tidying, but their home never stays tidy for long. This can lead to feelings of failure – *Everyone else can keep their home tidy* – or it can lead to arguments with their loved ones who, they often feel, are the reason their homes stay messy. These feelings are perfectly normal and felt by most people at one time or another.

Our home reflects our mind, and if our environment is chaotic, then so are our thoughts. Physical clutter leads to emotional clutter, and it's harder to maintain relationships when surrounded by mess. It is also difficult to focus on emotional conversations. Studies show, when we are in a messy environment, we have difficulty regulating emotions and are often reactive and easily irritated by others. Clutter increases the stress hormone, cortisol, which can affect our pulse and blood pressure. While it is healthy to have small amounts of cortisol, chronic high levels can lead to anxiety, depression and can affect our immune system, leaving our bodies susceptible to disease and illness.

A messy environment drains our energy and affects our sleep, and despite feeling fatigued, clients often report they have difficulty falling asleep at night. This has a knock-on effect the following day as it is difficult to have a productive day while feeling exhausted and sleep-deprived.

You can buy things that release serotonin and dopamine, the 'happy' hormones, which satisfies an emotional need and delights us momentarily, but this feeling soon wears off and the item sits at the back of the cupboard and is never used.

Everything we own has an emotion attached to it, and quite often it is easier to keep the item than deal with that emotion. We may dislike an item but keep it because it would be wasteful to let it go; after all, we spent good money on it. The sunk cost, however, is that as soon as we bought it, our money was gone.

Look at your present environment and consider how you feel. Do you feel relaxed and at ease or are you feeling unsettled and anxious? If it is the latter, and you are feeling dissatisfied with your current environment, that is good because you will be inspired for something better. Raymond Holliwell shared that, 'If you are working for success, look at the home; if order is the first law, then it must also be your first application.'

FINANCIAL

Our messy home costs us money! It can be tempting to buy extras when they are discounted, after all, we feel we are saving money, but this leads to stockpiling and bulging cupboards with duplicates of items we will never use. This was evident when organising my client's garage where we unearthed over £9,000 worth of excess tools, painting and gardening equipment. My client bought many of these items because he didn't know he already had them and others because they were a bargain. Imagine what he could have used this money for instead!

Disorganised paperwork has hidden costs, as vouchers and cheques are well out of date by the time we find them, and our mislaid bills cause us to accrue late fees for missing payments. We have to pay to replace anything we can't find, often buying duplicates of important documents and many of us are not aware we are still being charged for things we signed up to and no longer need.

Disorganisation and clutter in business has huge financial implications, causing money to continually leak like a dripping tap. With no clear organisation, we rebuy things because we can't find them, or we don't know we have them, and this extra cost soon adds up. When we sit in a messy work environment, our brain has to multitask, and we are unable to properly focus on a task. This leads to loss of productivity, lack of motivation and creativity. The physical effects of clutter can impact our health, leading to periods of sickness and time away from our desks.

Most of us can identify with the feeling of frustration at not being able to find what we are looking for, and clutter costs us precious time, with people in messy homes spending an average of forty minutes each day searching for items in their homes. Even when they're looking right at the lost item, it becomes difficult to see when surrounded by clutter. As busy people, we neither have the time, the inclination nor the energy to go through this every day. Once we organise and tidy, we find things effortlessly and enjoy more free time – a study found once this is completed, it takes 40% less time to clean our homes. That's a win-win for me.

MOVING FORWARD

Once we have made the decision to get started, we need to create an ideal vision.

I encourage my clients to spend twenty minutes in their favourite room, close their eyes and visualise their ideal day and how it would support their ideal lifestyle. I get them to consider how their home will support the person they aspire to be. Then they write this vision down in technicolour detail so that each time they read it, they will feel as though they are already living this.

This is so powerful, and in my opinion, the most important part of tidying. Having a clear image will keep us motivated, it will keep momentum going and be the driving factor pushing us towards your finish line. On those days we don't want to tidy, revisit our ideal life-style and remember our *why*.

When working with clients, I motivate and encourage them each step of the way so it may be beneficial for you to have an accountability buddy, someone who will cheer you on when you are making great progress and when your momentum dips. I suggest you set aside time each day to tidy; remain consistent and these small steps will get you towards the end goal of completion and satisfaction. If you want this strongly enough, you will do it.

POSITIVES

Tidying improves our mood, and we find joy in owning and caring for less. Once we organise our spaces, we know exactly what we have and where it is – so we don't need to re-buy. We let go of those items we don't need and give everything we are keeping a home. When we are finished using each item, we put it back in this place, and this simple concept makes it so easy to keep it tidy.

Cleaning materials, toiletries and make-up are three categories that most of us have excess of. I encourage my clients to only keep one or two of each item for current use, and create their own 'shop', a separate cupboard where they store those excess items together. They display them neatly, just as they would see in a supermarket. Then, when they need to replenish an item, they check their own shop before buying it again. This stops them overbuying and helps them use what they already have.

Clients are amazed by how much personal growth they have as they organise their home. They see several patterns emerge and begin to understand their previous shopping habits (whether they were a last-minute shopper or a bargain lover), style of clothes that they want to keep and that suit them, and they make a definite decision to shop mindfully in the future.

The tidying process allows for self-reflection and empowers us to make informed choices when we are ready to do so. When we surround ourselves with items we love, we feel amazing and want that feeling to last. We then start to hold everything else in our life to these same principles, and before long, we reassess relationships and friendships, gravitating towards people with similar interests and values as ourselves and setting exciting new goals in our life.

Once my clients spend the time and energy tidying their homes, they change their shopping habits. Now, that doesn't mean they won't shop again; however, it does encourage them to shop mindfully and only make that purchase if they love it or need it.

DECISION-MAKING

When we organise and tidy our home, we tidy by category, bringing similar items together. This allows us to see how many of each item we own and to realise we have enough already – this helps change our thoughts from lack to abundance.

We hold each item close to our heart and decide whether we love it or need it, and we only need to think about one item at a time, which takes the overwhelm out of this process. If you love it (or need it) then you keep it with confidence, and if it doesn't meet the mark, you thank it and let it go with gratitude.

When letting items go, it is important we don't feel guilty, as guilt is a toxic emotion. Indeed, a study by Professor Gates of Washington DC looked at the chemical reaction of guilt in our bodies and found it was akin to pouring acid on our body; it will seep into our skin and destroy. Instead, let these items go with gratitude, they came into our lives for a reason, so we should send them off with our thanks. When we have an attitude of gratitude, we are in a higher vibration and therefore attracting more of the same into our lives.

Making these small decisions when it doesn't really matter helps us become confident in our decision-making so we can easily make decisions when it really matters. As you tidy your home, you will hone your decision-making skills and become more confident about those difficult decisions. You begin to trust your intuition and learn what to place value on. We appreciate what we have, and rarely do we miss what we discarded.

VIBRATIONS

Clutter keeps us from living the life we deserve, and it stops us from achieving our ideal lifestyle. Consider how we feel when we enter a cluttered room. The energy in that room is stagnant and our vibrations and energies are low – this stagnant energy has no room to flow, and we adopt a pessimistic mindset. This is disempowering and prevents us from reaching our full potential.

When we avoid dealing with physical clutter, we avoid dealing with it emotionally and this energy becomes stuck. We hold this image constantly in our minds which lowers our vibrations. This also relates to those items that we cannot see, the unopened boxes in the attic or the contents of our bulging cupboards.

Organising and tidying our home is the first step towards living the life we deserve, our ideal lifestyle and the new us. It can be an emotional and spiritual journey, where we learn so much about ourselves and our dreams for the future. We learn how to select and cherish the belongings that make us *truly* happy, and we come to understand that nothing outside of us will ever equate to our worth inside. We realise we don't need to buy something to make us feel fulfilled – we know that *we* are enough.

Indeed, when we are not frantically rushing about and are more relaxed, we notice and appreciate all the beautiful items we own. This raises our vibrations and helps us attract more fabulous things into our life.

CONCLUSION

The return on investment of organising our homes and businesses is priceless. Completing our tidying will certainly free up precious time, and for every ten minutes spent decluttering, we can gain hours of our life back. We also see financial savings when we only buy what we need and love and then, of course, we have the wonderful benefits to our emotional and mental wealth.

Tidying is not just about decluttering our physical space; it's about achieving a home that we love and that brings joy into our life and harmony into our surroundings. The process is cathartic and helps us achieve an environment that soothes and quiets the mind, while building mental strength. As we become more tranquil, we gain deep inner peace.

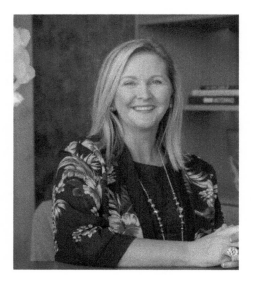

SHARON MC NULTY

A professional home and business organiser and founder of Joyful Spaces.

Maybe you've heard the old adage: tidy house, tidy mind?

Whether you know it or not, the space you live and work in significantly impacts your mood, productivity and mental wellbeing.

Maybe you've found yourself complaining you've nothing to wear, despite a wardrobe chock-a-block with clothes?

Perhaps you feel the urge to 'tidy' but haven't a clue where to start. And let's be honest, who's got the time?

Lucky for you – creating joyful spaces is what I do.

When you work with me, we'll transform your home or business by creating a space that works for you. If you're ready to bring peace, harmony and simplicity back into your life, you're in the right place.

And the good news? Using my method, it's a one-time job!

Not only will your physical space be calm and peaceful, but your mind will be too.

Are you ready to breathe easier and leave anxiety and guilt behind? To feel energised and motivated whilst finally having the house and space you dreamed of.

I know, I changed my own life this way.

Working as a midwife and health visitor, and mum of three, I was juggling all the balls, struggling to manage everything, and spent most weekends clearing up only to have to do it again midweek. It felt like a vicious cycle.

When I discovered Marie Kondo's book *The Life-Changing Magic of Tidying Up* in 2014 – something clicked. I studied under her and become a master consultant in the KonMari method.

Over the last eight years, I've appeared on TV and radio to discuss this work and have built a team who work internationally, changing lives by transforming spaces. Now, I want the same for you. Because let's be honest, we all deserve a little more joy!

We can work together one to one in-home or virtually to create a tailor-made plan, or I have a variety of online courses and workshops available if you're a fan of a bit of DIY.

Bottom line: when you work with me, you'll never have to feel frustrated by chaos again.

Instead, you can find genuine joy, peace and harmony in your surroundings and learn how to select and cherish the belongings that make you truly happy.

Let's make your space a joyful one.

NEVER THE
SAME AGAIN

Trevor Verner

There are nine children in my family, then Mum and Dad. So I have a family of eleven; six boys and three girls including my twin sister. We were the youngest for seven years until my little brother came along. As a child I was always drawing or doing scribbles on pieces of paper. I also loved listening to music, so any chance I got I would sit at the kitchen table with headphones on and draw. My mum was always very encouraging about the drawing, I think because one of her brothers enjoyed sketching – she always talked about his drawing.

My primary school teacher always got me to draw things up on the blackboard in class with chalk. If there were any posters to make, I was given the task to do them. It was great at the time because it made me feel important. I was never an academic pupil, I just enjoyed doing things with my hands like woodwork and metalwork. Cathy Cook was my art teacher in secondary school, and it was her who encouraged me to do my art because she felt I had a great talent in pencil drawing.

We were a very close family. As a boy growing up, I had a lovely childhood surrounded by my big brothers and sisters, and we had some special times as a family. Christmas, for me, was a really exciting time, there was always a great buzz in the build-up to the festive season. Mum was hard at work preparing for the celebrations. I loved the smell of home cooking, especially the smell of Christmas puddings and cake. The smell of baked cakes was in the air for weeks. School still played a part; we were making Christmas decorations for the assembly hall because they were giving the school a festive look.

My story really begins at Christmas, 1975. I was twelve years of age, a young boy wondering what life had in store for me, what adventures I would have. Little did I know that it was going to be the start of something traumatic and frightening – a dark time in my life

Christmas holidays from school had arrived. I was outside playing with my close friends who lived in my park. Christmas Eve had arrived, the atmosphere was amazing. We were all in such good form, the house was full of Christmas cheer – the colourful lights on the tree gave out such a warm glow. It was time for me to go to bed, but later that night my eldest brother, Ronnie, came up the stairs. He was in the bathroom when he called me and asked me to help him fasten a chain around his neck. As I put it on I asked him what it was. He said that it was a St Christopher that his girlfriend had got him and it was to keep him safe when travelling. He then said, 'Ted,' (that was a wee name he called me) 'you get back into bed, Santa's coming tonight.' He also said, 'I'll see you on Boxing Day.' He was going to work on night duty and also working on Christmas morning so that he could be off later. He was going to his girlfriend's house for Christmas afternoon.

Ronnie was such a nice person. I used to wash his car and do wee chores for him when I could. He would often get me to blow-dry his hair – we just had a very relaxed brotherly relationship.

Sleeping that night was so hard because I was thinking about Christmas morning. About six in the morning my sister and I woke and were so excited to see what Santa had left under the tree. We got our presents and Mum got up early to get the turkey on. With a big family to feed, she spent the whole morning doing jobs to make our Christmas dinner special. We played with our toys and also helped out with things getting ready for the big day that was ahead. The smells in the house were amazing, everybody was in good form, Christmas music playing in the background, it was just lovely.

Little did we know what trauma and devastation would be inflicted on us as a family later on that day. Dad was working so he was due home at four o'clock. The day was a real winter's day – it was raining, the fire was on, it was burning with hot coals making us feel snug and warm. My face was glowing, and we were all huddled around watching television. There was so much on that day. The highlight of the programs for me was the film *The Wizard of Oz*. I can remember so clearly. We were all sitting down on the floor, Dad had come home and he was resting comfortably in the chair. The lights in the house were down low, Mum had opened a box of sweets, the film had started, and we were well into the film when a knock came on the door. I remember Dad getting up and going into the hall. He closed the door and went to see who was there. We were still watching the film. He came into the room, put the light on straightaway and said, 'Ronnie has been in an accident, it's not good, bad accident.' For me, as a twelve-year-old boy, it felt that time had stopped, there and then.

Seeing all my brothers and sisters crying and Mum so distressed, I wanted to help but couldn't. I felt so helpless even at that age – my mind was in freefall; I didn't know how to react. One minute I was crying, the next I was staring silently wondering if Ronnie would be okay. I wasn't to know that this was really the start of my mental health being affected by a trauma.

Mum and Dad and the older members of the family went into the hospital to see Ronnie. I didn't go because I was scared, so my twin sister and I stayed with my next-door neighbour. It was a long evening; my mind was all over the place wondering what was going to happen. Later that night, the family came home. Ronnie had died in the early hours of Boxing Day. When coming home from work he had crashed his car and suffered a severe head injury due to being thrown out of the back window. Dad had to make the decision to have the life support machine switched off as Ronnie would never have made a full recovery. That must have been the most heart-wrenching thing for any mother or father to have to do for their child, no matter what age. Ronnie was only twenty-one.

There was, I felt, a real dark shadow that had fallen on the family. Everyone was so sad, people were crying. Mum kept a wee fire on that night. I remember hearing sobbing and yet times of quietness, obviously brothers and sisters deep in thought about Ronnie. Some of them went to bed but I know I got no sleep thinking about him. That next day was so hard, I had never seen my dad so upset. He had been so brave for everyone on Christmas Day, but he just broke down when we were all back home. It was so hard to listen to family members talking about Ronnie's funeral. This was so final – we were never going to see him again.

During that time I can remember people visiting us in the house. People just kept coming and talking to Mum and Dad and the rest of the family. I didn't get to go to his funeral because the youngest of us were kept away and were sent round to another neighbour's house. We were told it was a very big funeral, and people continued to call for days afterwards. Christmas was never the same again.

There was just this void. I missed Ronnie's big smile, his great sense of humour. He was my hero. He was so fit having been involved in so many sports – swimming, badminton, football and athletics were his favourites. It was just so hard to accept, even at twelve years of age, that Ronnie was gone.

The school holidays were over, and people were trying to get back to normal – whatever normal could be. When I went to school, teachers were saying how sorry they were about Ronnie. He was well-liked, and our family were well-known. School was hard for me because I couldn't concentrate in class.

My art was the only subject that I could lose myself in. I could let all the pain and sorrow out of my head. But when I came home, I could see and feel the sadness in the family. I tried to help Mum when I could, but she was so heartbroken. I was still so confused about it all. I knew Ronnie was gone but I couldn't express my feelings. I tried to ask questions about Ronnie but Mum found it hard to talk about it and I just felt so helpless. In that first year after his death, there was so many strange thoughts and ideas going through my mind, obviously in relation to Ronnie's death. I missed him so much. I worried about what it must have been like for him, it must have been so scary as he lay on the ground injured, was there no-one around to help him. It must have been so lonely on that road, yet he was only a few miles from home. All these thoughts were going through my mind all the time.

Mum tried to tell me about Ronnie because I found it hard to see his face in my mind. I often went upstairs to the boys' bedroom – in the cupboard mum had a few bits of Ronnie's clothes. I got comfort from smelling them to get his scent. She gave me a small photo of him, he was just as I remembered.

My life was hard from then on, I discovered through another significant event in my life that I was suffering from PTSD. This was a turning point for me. I left my job in the forces and decided to take time off to concentrate on getting better. You see, we all need time out sometimes to work on ourselves, discover who we are and what it is that improves and maintains our wellbeing. When you concentrate on being your best self then everything changes around you.

Having had a feeling of no self-worth for years, and then trying to build myself up – mind, body and soul – to where I was, I knew I could bring a lot of myself to this relationship with love, kindness and honesty. I knew that I was still going to have to protect my mental health, but I had confidence in myself to control things and work at it, and try not to let it damage my new life.

Meeting Gloria was a turning point for me, she helped me a lot and I gained in confidence and started to believe in myself. When Gloria and I met she already had two small boys, Ross and Peter, four and two. Having a lot of older brothers and sisters who were already married, I had quite a few nieces and nephews, so I was used to young children and liked being around them. So when I met the boys, I was able to embrace the whole situation and enjoyed being a part of the family. Gloria's help, support, kindness, love and commitment helped me not to feel vulnerable, but very special. I got to love Gloria and the boys, this gave me the drive to try and better myself.

This was such a turnaround from having no self-worth. I moved in with Gloria after about a year and we became a family. Soon after I moved in, I lost my job and had to change direction yet again. Gloria and I got talking about the things that inspired me, and we tried to make a link between the kind of things I could do for work and the things I enjoyed doing. We came up with a few ideas. I knew art and sport were going to be there, because I was still doing the things I had to do to protect my mental health. Whatever I decided to look at, it needed to be something that I liked doing, that I could be in control of, and that would be stimulating for my mental health. Gloria encouraged me to consider self-employment so that I could have a day job at something active, and then keep my art as a way to relax in the evenings and work towards an exhibition. We decided on me taking the plunge to become a self-employed painter and decorator, as I had learned something about the trade when I was younger in a part-time job. This was such a big decision for me because it was something hopefully that I could do for many years and keep my art running alongside. I looked into the process of getting started, and got help from a business startup scheme. I couldn't have imagined a few years earlier that I would be starting my own business and have the confidence to make a new life for myself.

A few more years passed, we were blessed with a boy Daniel, and soon after we had the good news that our fourth child was on the way. We had a lovely healthy wee girl – we called her Grace. This for me was now the perfect family. It was a lovely feeling having a wonderful family and Gloria, my wife, who was so supportive of what I was doing.

However, things didn't always go smoothly, and I had various spells of anxiety and still had flashbacks and nightmares. For years I used to get so angry in the weeks coming up to Christmas, about anything and nothing, and we just rode the storm – but it wasn't doing anybody any good. As the kids got older they began to watch out for my change of mood. Eventually Gloria suggested that we make an effort to include something tangible to remember all our lost loved ones at Christmas, including Ronnie and Gloria's sister Robena – who had died more recently – and her dad. Gloria suggested lighting candles for each of them, such a simple thing, but I find it gives me a focus as if they are with us, so we as a family light them on Christmas Day and Boxing Day, and I find that very calming. Christmas became something to look forward to again. Finding what works for you is so important, especially for your wellbeing. This ritual has taken the pain away somewhat and allowed us to enjoy family time again.

I now build on my decorating business and carry on with my artwork. I want to develop my skills further and try to have more exhibitions professionally. I have hosted many exhibitions now and they have gone very well so I was excited to keep going. I found this easy to do because my passion was with art and again it was all helping my mental health. I can honestly say that it never felt like work. I am so lucky being able to do something that I love and when I come home after a day's work I am not even stressed. I am in control, protecting my mental health and wellbeing which I work on every day.

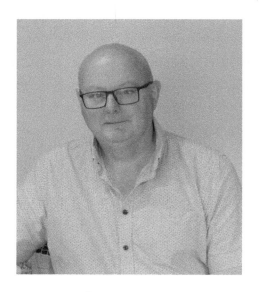

TREVOR VERNER

Trevor Verner is an artist and art therapy tutor who lives with his wife and family in Ballinamallard, Co Fermanagh.

Trevor has been a professional artist for thirty-five years, his medium is pencil.

He has had nineteen exhibitions – some solo and some with other artists.

This is a memoir of Trevor's journey with mental illness and recovery and his efforts to bring his art out into the community to help other people.

Trevor says, 'Working so much with my art and knowing the benefits it has for mental health, I decided fifteen years ago to take a program out into the community. I was lucky to get the opportunity to work with all different types of groups and using my program to change lives in mental health. I have now worked in many areas of mental health and I hope to continue to help people.'